10 DAY DIET

Quick and Easy Recipes for Weight loss, Detox your Body and Boost your Energy

ASHLEY David

Table of Contents

Introduction

Whether your weight-loss goals entail attempting to lose 5 pounds or more than 50, the very same concepts identify just how much weight you shed and just how quick your weight management will certainly take place. Bearing in mind the adhering to basic healthy and balanced consuming diet tips and also putting them right into technique can bring about weight reduction without the help of any special diet regimen plans, weight management programs, physical fitness books, or medications.

Our body weight is identified by the amount of power that we absorb as food and also the amount of energy we use up in the activities of our day. Power is determined in calories. Metabolic process is the amount of all chemical processes within the body that sustain life. Your basal metabolic price is the number of calories (amount of power) you need for your body to execute necessary functions. If your weight stays continuous, this is likely an indicator that you are absorbing the very same quantity of calories that you shed daily. If you're gradually gaining weight over time, it is likely that your caloric intake is greater than the variety of calories you melt through your day-to-day tasks.

Every adult is in control of the amount of food he or she consumes daily, so our intake of calories is something we can regulate. To a major level, we can additionally control our output of energy, or the variety of calories we shed daily. The variety of calories we melt every day depends on the following:

Our basic metabolic rate (BMR), the number of calories we shed per hr simply by being alive and also maintaining body functions

Our degree of exercise

For some people, because of genetic (acquired) factors or various other health conditions, the resting metabolic rate (RMR) can be slightly greater or lower than average. Our weight likewise contributes in figuring out the amount of calories we melt at rest-- the much more calories are required to keep your body in its present state, the better your body weight. A 100-pound individual requires much less power (food) to maintain body weight than an individual who weighs 200 pounds.

Way of life and job practices partly figure out the number of calories we need to consume daily. A person whose job involves heavy physical labor will normally shed more calories in a day than somebody who rests at a desk most of the day (a sedentary work). For people who do not have tasks that need extreme physical activity, workout or raised physical activity can enhance the variety of calories shed.

As a harsh estimate, a typical woman 31-50 years old who leads an inactive way of life requires regarding 1,800 calories daily to preserve a regular weight. A guy of the same age needs regarding 2,200 calories. Taking part in a modest level of physical activity (exercising 3 to 5 days weekly) calls for concerning 200 additional calories daily.

CHAPTER 1

15 Ways to Motivate Yourself to Lose Weight:

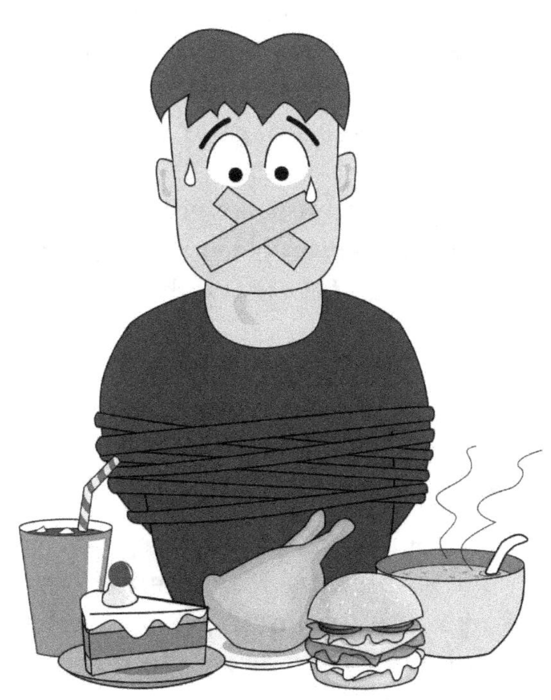

Sticking and also beginning to a healthy and balanced weight management plan can sometimes appear impossible.

Frequently, people simply lack the motivation to begin or lose their motivation to keep going. Thankfully, motivation is something you can work to raise.

This post talks about 16 ways to encourage yourself to drop weight.

1. Determine Why You Intend To Slim Down

Plainly specify all the reasons you want to reduce weight as well as create them down. This will certainly help you stay dedicated as well as inspired to reach your weight loss objectives.

Attempt to review them daily and use them as a suggestion when tempted to wander off from your fat burning strategies.

Your factors might include protecting against diabetic issues, keeping up with grandchildren, looking your best for an event, enhancing your positive self-image or suitable right into a specific set of pants.

Many individuals begin dropping weight due to the fact that their doctor suggested it, yet research study reveals that individuals are much more successful if their weight loss motivation comes from within

Recap: Plainly define your weight management goals and compose them down. See to it your motivation is driven from within for long-lasting success.

2. Have Practical Assumptions

Numerous diet regimens and also diet regimen products assert very easy and quick fat burning. Nonetheless, most professionals suggest only losing 1-- 2 extra pounds (0.5-- 1 kg) per week

Setting unattainable goals can bring about sensations of irritation and trigger you to surrender. As a matter of fact, setting and also achieving attainable objectives causes feelings of achievement.

Likewise, individuals who reach their self-determined weight reduction objectives are most likely to preserve their fat burning lasting

A study utilizing data from numerous weight management centers located that females who anticipated to lose one of the most weight were the most likely to leave of the program

The bright side is that just a little weight loss of 5-- 10% of your body weight can have a large influence on your wellness. If you are 180 pounds (82 kg), that is simply 9-- 18 pounds (4-- 8 kg). It's 13-- 25 pounds (6-- 11 kg) if you are 250 extra pounds (113 kg).

Actually, losing 5-- 10% of your body weight can:.

- Enhance blood sugar control.
- Decrease the danger of cardiovascular disease.
- Reduced cholesterol degrees.
- Decrease joint discomfort.
- Decrease the threat of specific cancers.

Recap: Establish realistic weight-loss expectations to increase feelings of accomplishment as well as prevent stress out. Just a modest quantity of weight-loss of 5-- 10% can have a significant influence on your health and wellness.

3. Concentrate On Refine Goals.

Many individuals trying to lose weight only established end result objectives, or objectives they wish to achieve at the end.

Normally, an outcome objective will be your last target weight.

However, focusing only on outcome goals can derail your motivation. They can typically feel also far-off and also leave you feeling overwhelmed.

Instead, you must set process objectives, or what actions you're going to take to reach your desired end result. An example of a process objective is exercising four times a week.

A research study in 126 obese women participating in a weight loss program found those who were process concentrated were most likely to slim down as well as less likely to deviate from their diet regimens, contrasted to those that focused on fat burning end results alone.

Consider setting SMART objectives to set strong objectives. WISE

represent:.
- Specific.
- Quantifiable.
- Attainable.
- Realistic.
- Time-based.
Some examples of SMART objectives consist of:.
- I will certainly stroll quickly for thirty minutes five days following week.
- I will certainly eat 4 portions of vegetables each day this week.
- I will only consume alcohol one soda today.
Recap: Setting WISE procedure objectives will certainly help you stay motivated, while focusing only on end result objectives can bring about frustration as well as lower your motivation.

4. Pick a Plan That Fits Your Lifestyle.

Find a weight reduction plan that you can adhere to, and also stay clear of plans that would certainly be almost impossible to adhere to in the long term.

While there are numerous various diets, the majority of are based on reducing calories.

Lowering your calorie consumption will result in weight reduction, but diet programs, especially frequent yo-yo dieting, has actually been discovered to be a forecaster of future weight gain.

Therefore, avoid stringent diets that totally eliminate specific foods. Research has discovered that those with an "all or absolutely nothing" frame of mind are much less most likely to slim down.

Instead, think about creating your own personalized strategy. The complying with dietary habits have actually been verified to assist you slim down:.
- Lowering calorie consumption.
- Minimizing part sizes.
- Reducing frequency of snacks.
- Reducing fried food as well as desserts.
- Including vegetables and fruits.

Recap: Select an eating plan that you can stay with long term and also avoid extreme or quick-fix diet plans.

5. Maintain a Weight Reduction Journal.

Self-monitoring is critical to weight loss inspiration and also success.

Research has located that people that track their food consumption are more likely to lose weight as well as keep their weight reduction.

Nonetheless, to maintain a food journal properly, you have to document everything you consume. This includes dishes, snacks and the piece of sweet you consumed off your colleague's desk.

You can likewise tape your feelings in your food journal. This can aid you determine certain triggers for eating way too much and help you discover much healthier methods to cope.

You can keep food journals on pen and paper or use a website or application. They have all been confirmed efficient.

Recap: Maintaining a food journal can assist you measure progression, determine triggers and also hold yourself responsible. You can utilize a site or application as a device for monitoring as well.

6. Celebrate Your Successes.

Slimming down is hard, so celebrate all your successes to keep yourself motivated.

Give yourself some credit rating when you complete an objective.

Social media or weight-loss sites with community pages are wonderful places to share your successes as well as obtain support.

You will increase your motivation when you feel satisfaction in yourself.

Additionally, remember to celebrate behavior adjustments and also not simply getting to a particular number on the scale.

For instance, if you satisfied your goal of exercising 4 days a week, take a bubble bathroom or strategy an enjoyable evening with buddies.

Furthermore, you can additionally boost your motivation by gratifying yourself.

However, it is essential to choose appropriate benefits. Prevent gratifying on your own with food. Additionally, prevent rewards that are so expensive you would never buy it, or so irrelevant that you would enable yourself to have it anyway.

The following are some examples of incentives:.

- Obtaining a manicure.
- Going to a film.
- Acquiring a new running top.
- Taking a cooking course.

Recap:

Commemorate all your successes throughout your fat burning trip. Consider rewarding on your own to additionally increase your motivation.

7. Find Social Support.

People require routine assistance and also positive responses to remain determined.

Tell your close family and friends about your weight management objectives so they can assist sustain you on your journey.

Lots of people likewise discover it handy to find a fat burning friend. You can exercise together, hold each other liable and motivate each other throughout the process.

Additionally, it can be practical to include your companion, yet make certain to get assistance from other individuals also, such as your buddies.

In addition, think about signing up with a support system. Both online and in-person support groups have been verified to be beneficial.

RECAP: Having solid social support will certainly assist hold you responsible as well as maintain you encouraged to drop weight. Consider joining a support group to assist enhance your inspiration along the road.

8. Make a Dedication.

Research study shows that those who make a public commitment are most likely to follow up with their objectives.

Informing others regarding your fat burning objectives will aid you remain answerable. Inform your close family and friends, and also take into consideration sharing them on social networks. The even more individuals you share your objectives with, the better the responsibility.

In addition, consider buying a fitness center membership, bundle of exercise courses or paying for a 5K beforehand. You are most likely to follow up if you have actually currently made an investment.

Recap: Making a public commitment to slim down will help you remain determined and also hold you responsible.

9. Believe and Talk Positively.

People who have favorable assumptions and feel confident in their capability to attain their goals have a tendency to lose more weight.

Likewise, people who make use of "modification talk" are more likely to follow up with strategies.

Change talk is making declarations regarding dedication to behavioral modifications, the factors behind them and the actions you will certainly take or are requiring to reach your objectives.

Consequently, start speaking favorably regarding your weight loss. Additionally, discuss the steps you are going to take and commit your thoughts out loud.

On the other hand, research study reveals that individuals who spend a lot of time only thinking concerning their dream weight are much less most likely to reach their goal. This is called emotionally delighting.

Rather, you must emotionally comparison. To emotionally comparison, invest a couple of minutes envisioning reaching your objective weight and after that spend another couple of mins visualizing any type of feasible challenges that might obstruct.

A research in 134 students had them mentally delight or emotionally contrast their dieting objectives. Those who emotionally contrasted were more probable to take action. They consumed fewer calories, worked out even more and consumed fewer high-calorie foods.

As seen in this study, mentally contrasting is more inspiring and causes extra action than psychologically delighting, which can trick your mind right into believing you have actually already been successful and also create you to never take any type of action to reach your goals.

Recap: Assume as well as talk positively concerning your weight reduction objectives, however ensure you are practical and also focus on the steps you must take to reach them.

10. Prepare for Obstacles as well as challenges.

Day-to-day stressors will certainly always turn up. Discovering methods to plan for them as well as creating correct coping abilities will help you remain determined regardless of what life tosses your method.

There will constantly be birthday celebrations, parties or vacations to attend. And there will constantly be stressors at the office or with family members.

It is necessary to start issue addressing as well as brainstorming about these possible weight reduction difficulties as well as setbacks. This will certainly maintain you from leaving track and also losing motivation.

Lots of people rely on food for comfort. This can swiftly bring about them deserting their weight-loss objectives. Producing proper coping abilities will stop this from occurring to you.

In fact, researches have actually shown that people who are better at managing stress and also have better coping approaches will certainly lose even more weight as well as keep it off longer.

Consider using a few of these techniques to handle stress:.

- Exercise.
- Technique square breathing.
- Wash.
- Go outside and obtain some fresh air.
- Call a good friend.
- Request help.

Remember to likewise plan for vacations, gatherings and dining in restaurants. You can research restaurant food selections beforehand and locate a healthy choice. At celebrations, you can bring a healthy and balanced meal or consume smaller sized portions.

RECAP: It is crucial to prepare for troubles and also have great coping techniques. If you use food as a coping device, start practicing various other means to deal.

11. Don't Go For Perfection as well as Forgive Yourself.

You do not need to be excellent to drop weight.

If you have an "all or nothing" approach, you're much less likely to attain your goals.

When you are too restrictive, you may find yourself claiming "I had a burger and also fries for lunch, so I might too have pizza for dinner." Instead, try to say, "I had a large lunch, so I should go for a healthier supper".

And prevent beating on your own up when you make a mistake. Self-defeating thoughts will certainly just prevent your inspiration.

Rather, forgive yourself. Bear in mind that one blunder is not going to ruin your development.

Recap: When you aim for perfection, you will rapidly lose your inspiration. By permitting yourself versatility and also forgiving yourself, you can remain motivated throughout your fat burning journey.

12. Discover to Love as well as Appreciate Your Body.

Study has repeatedly discovered that individuals who dislike their bodies are less likely to lose weight.

Taking actions to improve your body picture can assist you shed more weight and also maintain your weight loss.

Additionally, individuals who have a better body picture are more probable to select a diet plan they can endure and also attempt brand-new activities that will certainly help them reach their goals.

The complying with tasks can aid enhance your body image:.
- Workout.
- Value what your body can do.
- Do something for yourself, such as getting a massage therapy or manicure.
- Surround on your own with favorable people.
- Stop comparing on your own to others, especially versions.
- Wear garments you like which fit you well.
- Look in the mirror as well as say the things you like regarding yourself out loud.
Recap: Boosting your body photo can assist you stay encouraged to slim down. Try the tasks mentioned above to enhance your body picture.

13. Locate a Workout You Delight in.

Exercise is an integral part of reducing weight. Not only does it assist you shed calories, but it additionally enhances your wellness. The most effective kind is exercise you appreciate as well as can stay with.

There are many different types and also ways to exercise, and also it's important to discover various options to discover one you take pleasure in.

Take into consideration where you want to work out. Do you favor to be within or outdoors? Would certainly you instead work out at a fitness center or in the convenience of your own residence?

Additionally, identify if you choose to exercise alone or with a team. Team classes are incredibly popular, and they aid lots of people remain inspired. However, if you don't appreciate group courses, working out by yourself is equally as excellent.

Finally, pay attention to music while you exercise, as doing so can raise inspiration. Individuals additionally tend to work out longer when listening to music.

Recap: Workout not only helps you melt calories, it likewise makes you feel better. Discover an exercise you take pleasure in, so it can easily enter into your routine.

14. Discover a Role Model.

Having a role model can help you stay inspired to reduce weight. Nevertheless, you need to pick the appropriate sort of good example to maintain on your own motivated.

Hanging a picture of a cover girl on your refrigerator will not encourage you with time. Rather, locate a good example that you can conveniently associate with.

Having a relatable and also favorable role model may aid maintain you motivated.

Maybe you recognize a close friend who has actually shed a lot of weight and can be your ideas. You can also seek inspiring blogs or tales about people who have actually efficiently reduced weight.

Recap: Discovering a good example will help maintain you motivated. It is necessary to locate a good example that you can associate with.

15. Get a Pet.

Canines can be the perfect weight-loss companions. As a matter of fact, research studies show that having a canine can aid you drop weight.

First, pet dogs can raise your exercise.

A Canadian research study in pet owners found that individuals who had canines strolled an average of 300 mins per week, while people that did not have pet dogs just strolled approximately 168 minutes each week.

Second, pet dogs are great social support. Unlike your human exercise buddy, pet dogs are often excited to obtain some exercise.

As an included bonus offer, pet possession is shown to enhance total wellness and health. It has been linked to lower cholesterol, lower blood pressure and also decreased sensations of loneliness as well as clinical depression.

Recap: Canines possession can assist you reduce weight by enhancing your exercise as well as providing terrific social assistance in the process.

CHAPTER 2

recipes for your 10 day green
smoothie cleanse

These core smoothie recipes for your 10 day green smoothie cleanse are designed to detox your body, lose weight and boost energy. The shopping lists provided contain all the ingredients you need to make these delicious and healthy smoothies. You can be creative if you want to AFTER the detox. It's better to stick with these recipes as much as you can to lose 10 pounds in 10 days. Plus, they taste great to keep you motivated throughout the detox.

IMPORTANT: If you have a full-sized blender like Blendtec or Vitamix, you can easily make 2 liters of smoothie. If it's smaller, you need to divide the recipe and blend twice to make your smoothie for the whole day.

Now, let's get started!

Day 1: Green Lemonade Smoothie

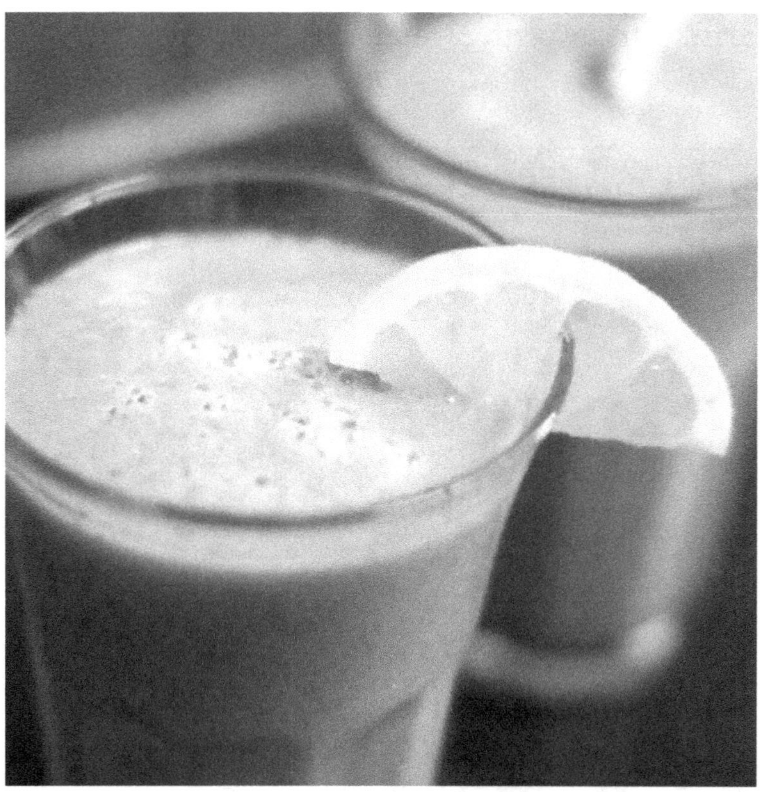

Green lemonade offers many health benefits. You will be delighted to know that it not only helps you in losing weight but it also keeps your heart healthy. Apples contain compounds that delay the breakdown of LDL i.e. bad cholesterol. Lemons help in boosting the immune system and reducing weight. Greens such as spinach, mint, kale, collard, coriander, chard etc. are also very beneficial for your health, especially spinach because it is rich in potassium, iron, fiber, lutein and folate.

Ingredients:

1) A peeled lemon
2) 2 green apples
3) 2 handfuls spinach or any other green mentioned above

Blend and drink this amazing weight loss smoothie.

Day 2: Green Detox Smoothie

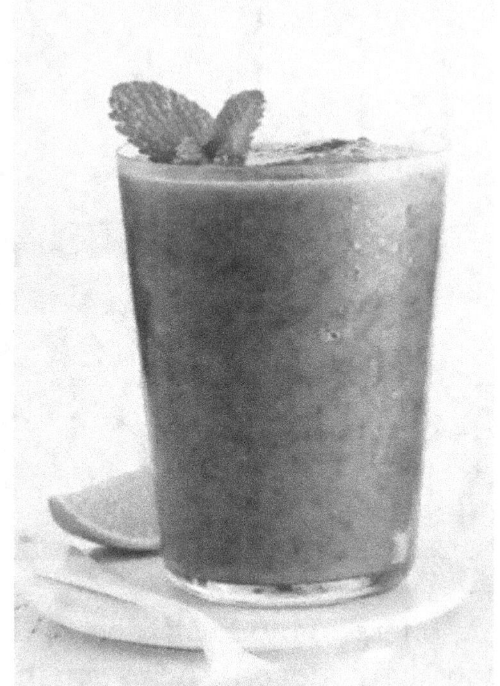

This smoothie contains a variety of greens. So, it's rich in iron and anti-oxidants. Plus, the high fiber content of this smoothie will help with constipation and weight loss.

Ingredients:

1) Fresh chopped mint – 1/4 cup
2) Chopped kale leaves – 1/4 cup
3) Chopped parsley – 1/4 cup
4) 2 chopped celery
5) Fresh orange juice – 1 cup
6) Mango cubes – 1 cup

Blend them nice and smooth and keep sipping this healthy and delicious green smoothie the entire day.

Day 3: Kale and Ginger Smoothie

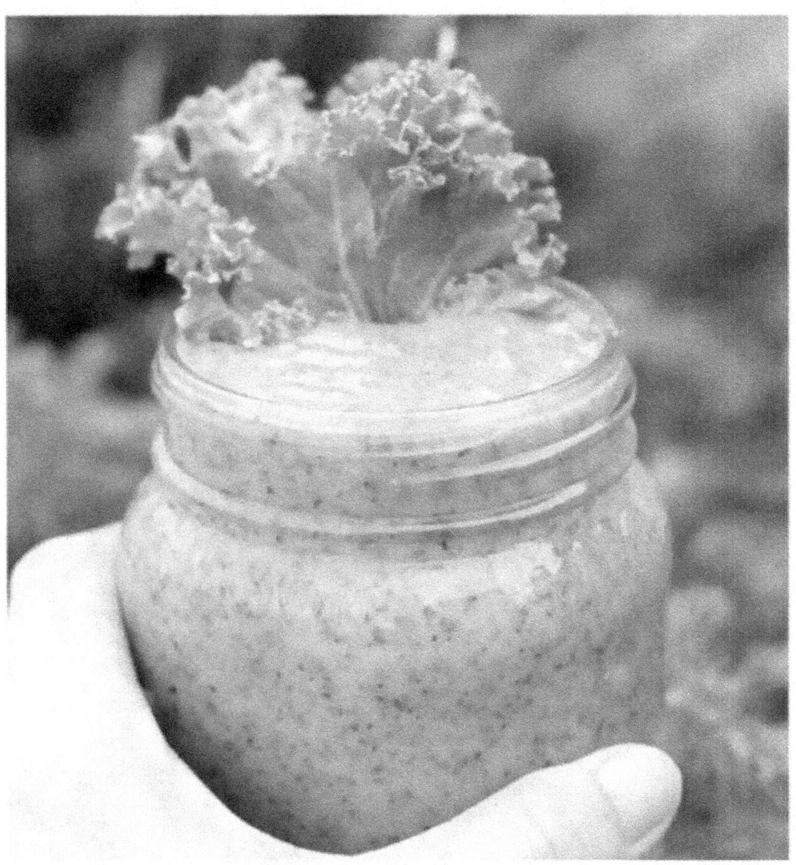

Kale and ginger is a superb combination. Kale has so much to offer for your health and ginger aids in digestion. Let's give it a go for our third day!

Ingredients:

1) Kale – 1 cup
2) Ginger – half inch

3) 1/4 avocado
4) Half cucumber
5) Half lemon
6) Coconut water – 1/2 cup
7) Water

Put everything in a blender, give it a whirl and you have a tasty and healthy green smoothie.

Day 4: Fresh Cucumber Smoothie

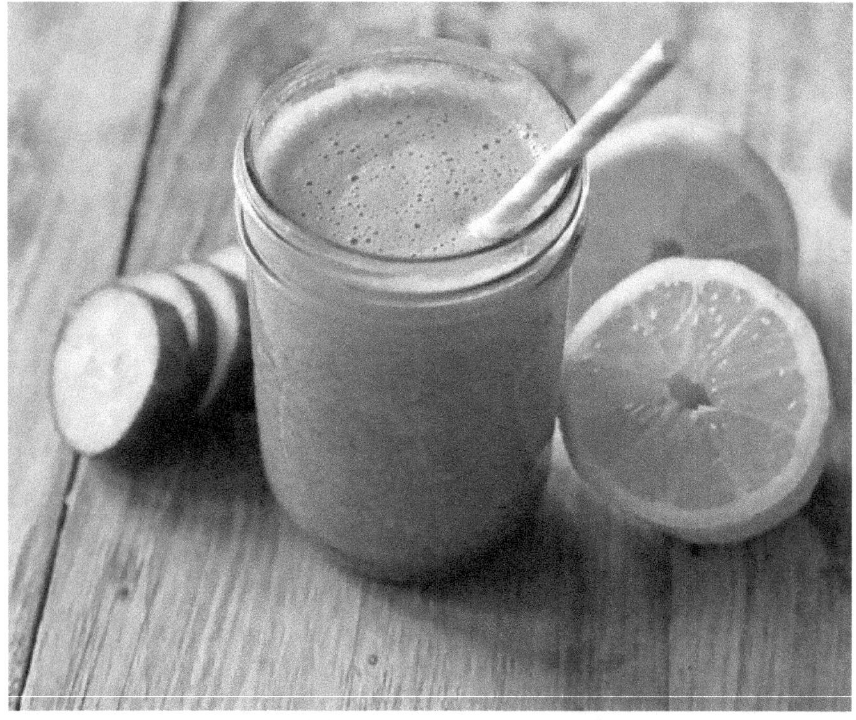

Making cucumber the base of your smoothie is a wise choice. It makes a good combination with leafy greens and keeps you hydrated throughout the day.

Ingredients:

1) 1 Cucumber
2) A fistful of kale
3) A fistful of romaine
4) 2 stalks of celery
5) 1 green apple
6) Half peeled lemon

Make a nice smoothie and freshen up each time you drink.

Day 5: Scrumptious Grape Smoothie

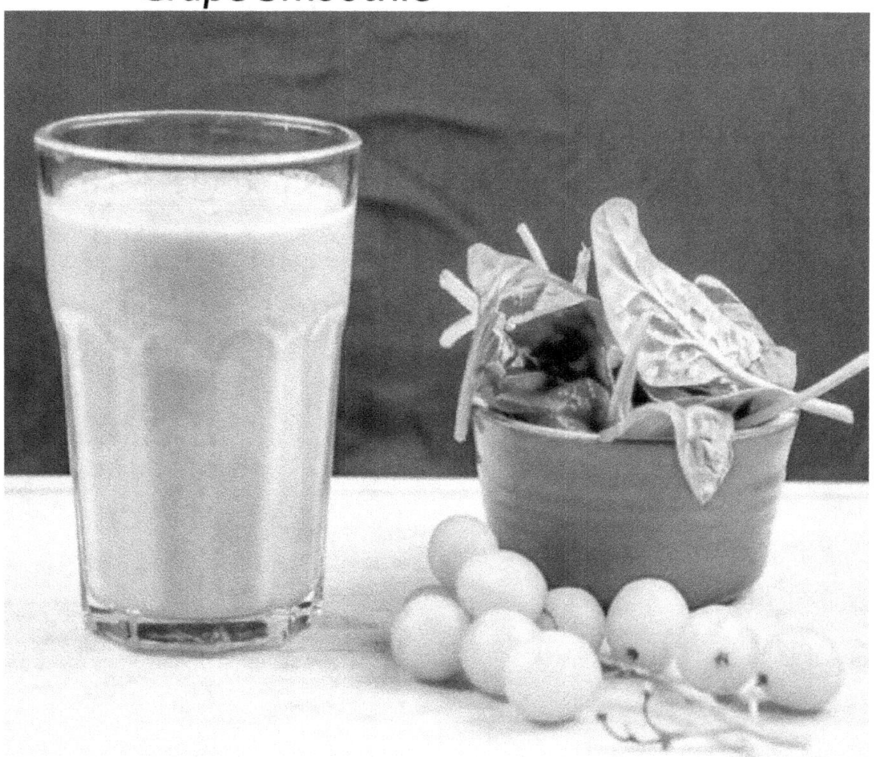

Grapes are not just mouth-watering, they pack so much energy when combined with kale and spinach. Adding other fruits like banana, orange and pear gives it a nice fruity flavor. You will enjoy it on the fifth day of detox.

Ingredients:

1) Green grapes – 1 cup
2) Spinach – 1 cup
3) Kale – 1 cup
4) A pear with its seeds, core and stem removed
5) 1 banana
6) 1 orange
7) Chia seeds – 1 tsp
8) ½ cup of water
9) Ice – 1/2 cup

Put all the ingredients in your blender and blend at slow speed for about 20 seconds. Then move to medium and high speed within the next 60 seconds. In less than 2 minutes, you'll have yourself a wonderful green smoothie.

Day 6: Amazing Spinach and Strawberry Smoothie

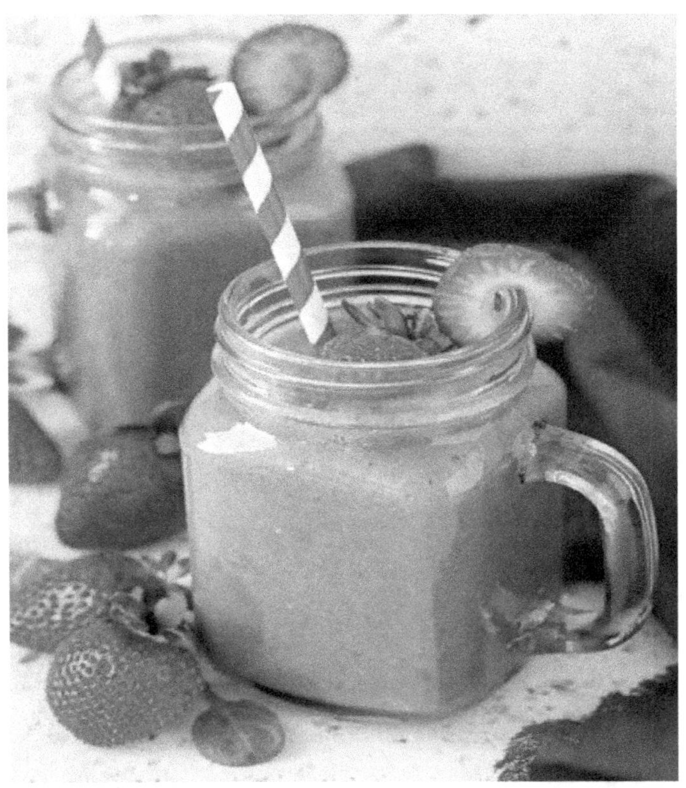

Add some twist in this classic spinach smoothie by adding strawberries and orange. Also, boost your metabolism by adding almond milk.

Ingredients:

1) Raw Spinach – 1 cup
2) Strawberries – 1/3 cup
3) 1 orange
4) Almond milk – 1 cup

Blend everything to a nice and smooth consistency.

Day 7: Spinach and Kale Smoothie

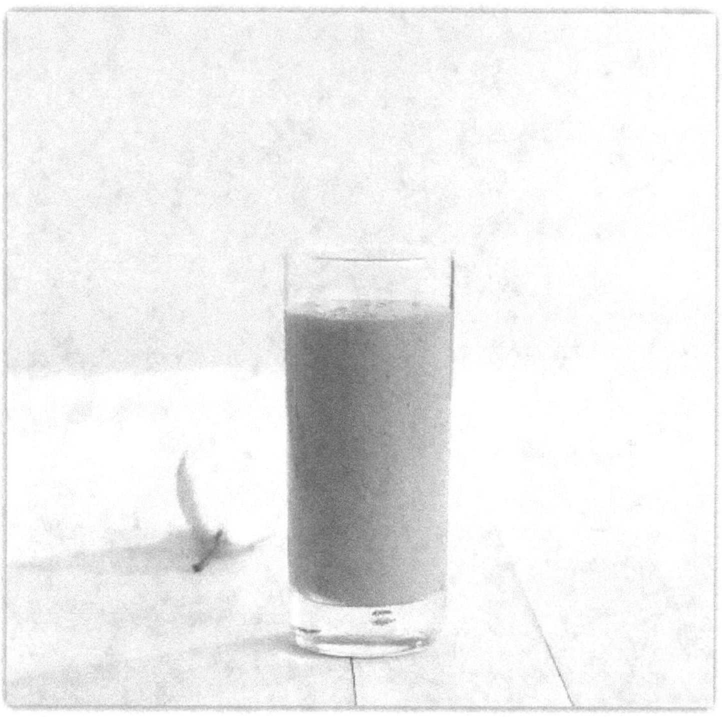

The goal of drinking these smoothies is not just losing weight. You need to look fresh and let me tell you the secret behind gorgeous skin – kale! It's full of carotenoids which gives your skin a healthy touch and makes it glow. Not only that, it also protects your skin from wrinkles. Drinking this smoothie is a perfect way to make your skin glow while you lose weight. Adding fruits like banana, grapes, pear and orange enhance the flavor and make you feel amazing throughout the day.

Ingredients:
1) Spinach – 1cup
2) Kale – 1 cup
3) Green grapes – 1cup
4) 1 orange

5) 1 pear
6) 1 banana
7) Chia seeds – 1 tsp
8) Water – half cup
9) Ice – 1/2 cup

Chop kale, spinach and pear. Blend them first and then add the rest of the ingredients and blend on high speed. Enjoy your smoothie!

Day 8: Pineapple Smoothie

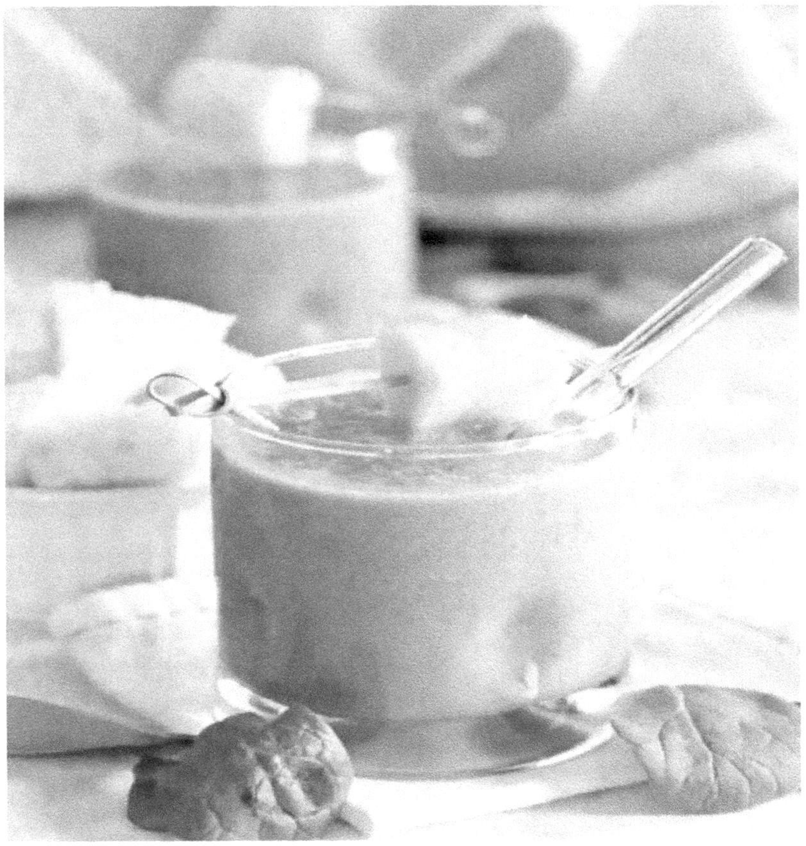

You see the bright green color of this pineapple smoothie comes from spinach. It is full of vitamin C because of pineapple and orange. Pineapple is also rich in manganese, folate and copper. A plant compound called bromelain is found in pineapples. It has so many benefits such as improved digestion, fighting cancer, healing properties and better immunity.

Ingredients:

1) Pineapple – 1/4 cup
2) Spinach – 1 cup
3) 1 orange
4) Almond milk – 1 cup

Blending these super healthy ingredients will be very useful for you for the whole day.

Day 9: Sweet Mango Cucumber Smoothie

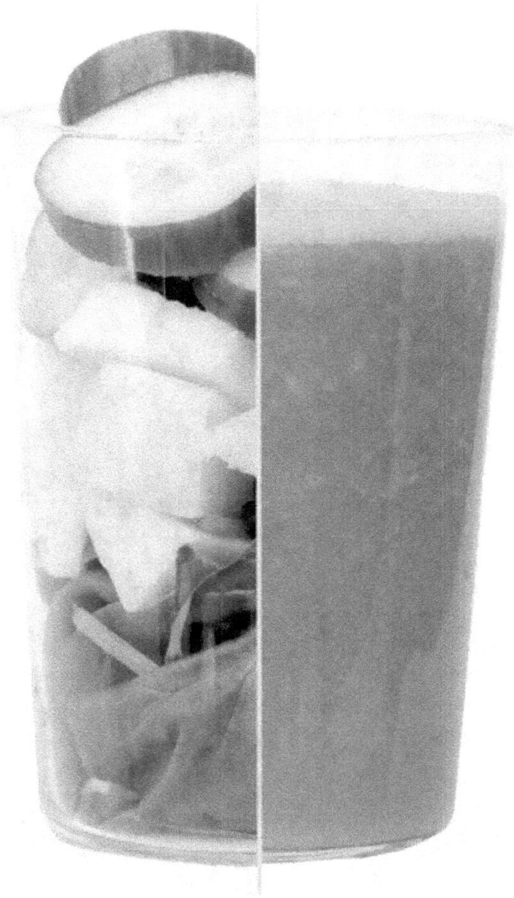

Here you have a very delicious mango cucumber smoothie. Thanks to the mangoes, you've got great flavor and lots of vitamins!

Ingredients:

1) Mangoes – 1/4 cup
2) Chopped Cucumber – 1 cup
3) 1 orange
4) Flaxseed – 1 tbsp.
5) Spinach – 1 cup

Make a smooth drink and stay fresh!

Day 10: Kale and Blueberry Smoothie

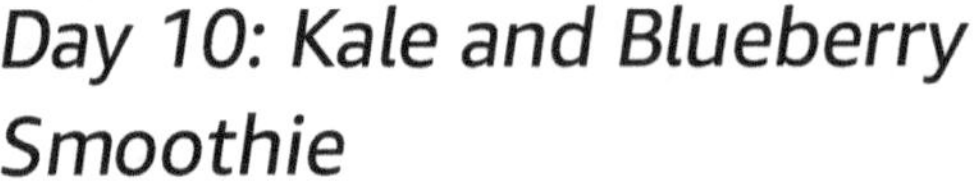

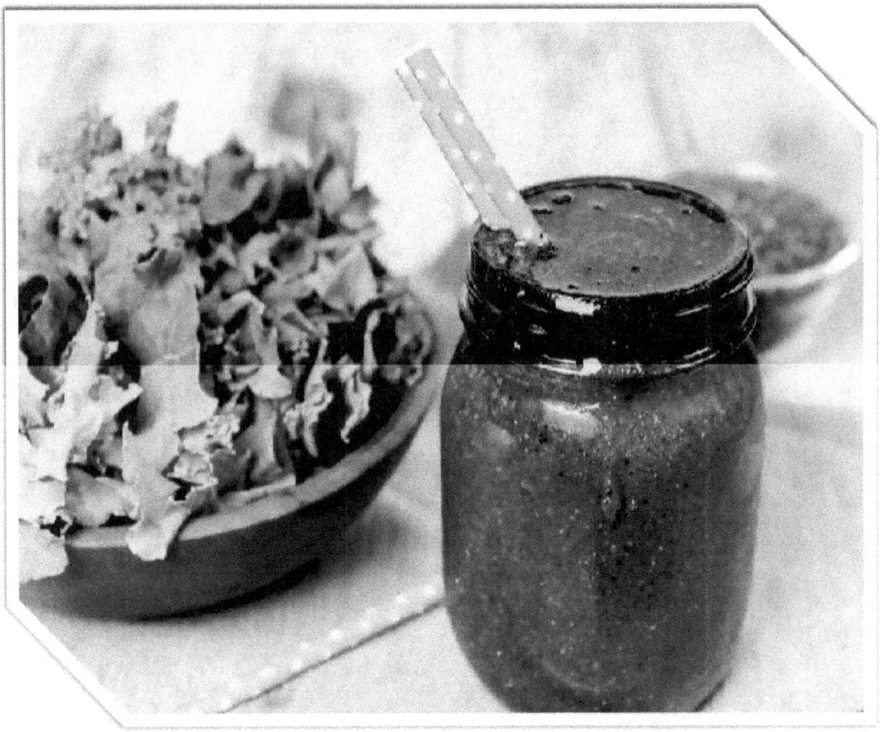

This is called hiding your greens and making it appealing for the whole family. The dark color of blueberries will hide kale and you will love the flavor. You will get antioxidants from blueberries and cherries. Kale, on the other hand, is pretty amazing because it has very few calories. Besides helping you to lose weight, it has loads of vitamin C which will boost your immunity.

Ingredients:

1) Kale – 1 cup
2) Blueberries – 1/2 cup

3) Cherries – 1/2 cup
4) Honey – 2 tsp
5) Almond milk – 1 cup

Make a creamy and tasty smoothie out of these amazing ingredients.

Best wishes for these 10 important days of your life. Try to include smoothies even after the detox in your daily routine. This will be helpful for you and your family in maintaining a healthy lifestyle. Drink these smoothies and see for yourself what a drink of green veggies and fruits can do for you. Your goal should not be to look "perfect". You will lose weight but the most important part is that you should *feel healthy*.

CHAPTER 3

10 Day Walking Can Help You Lose Weight and Belly Fat

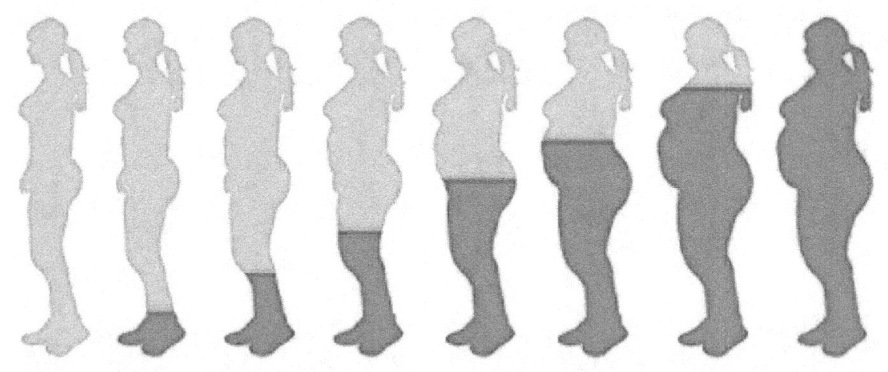

Due to the fact that being physically active decreases your risk of creating wellness problems like heart illness, diabetic issues and also cancer cells, this is Along with assisting you live a longer as well as much healthier life, exercise can likewise be beneficial for weight reduction and upkeep. The good news is, walking is a fantastic type of physical activity that's free, reduced danger as well as available to lots of people. Actually, walking isn't just great for you-- it's one of the most convenient forms of workout to incorporate into your day-to-day life. This post discovers just how strolling more often can assist you slim down as well as belly fat.

Walking Burns Calories

Your body needs power (in the form of calories) for all the complex chain reaction that enable you to relocate, breathe, think and also work generally. Nonetheless, daily calorie requirements vary from one person to another and are affected by points like your weight, sex, genes and task degree.It's well known that you need to shed more calories than you take in to drop weight. In addition, people that are more literally energetic melt even more calories. Nonetheless, modern-day living and also workplace might indicate that you spend large parts of your day sitting, particularly if you have an office job. Regrettably, a less active way of living can not only contribute to weight gain, it can likewise increase your danger of illness.

Trying to obtain even more workout by walking regularly can help you melt more calories and also reduce these dangers. In fact, strolling a mile (1.6 kilometres) burns about 100 calories, depending on your sex and also weight. One research gauged the variety of calories shed by non-athletes that walked at a quick rate of 3.2 miles (5 km) per hour or went for a pace of 6 mph for concerning a mile. It found those that walked at a quick speed melted an average of 90 calories per mile. In addition, although running burned significantly extra calories, it just melted around 23 more calories per mile, on average, suggesting both types of exercise added significantly to the variety of calories burned. To enhance the intensity of your walk and also burn even more calories, attempt walking on courses with hills or small inclines.

Recap: Walking burns calories, which might help you drop

weight and also maintain it off. As a matter of fact, strolling simply one mile burns regarding 100 calories.

It Aids Preserve Lean Muscle Mass

They usually shed some muscular tissue in enhancement to body fat when people reduced calories and also lose weight. This can be counterproductive, as muscle is a lot more metabolically energetic than fat. This suggests it helps you burn extra calories each day. Exercise, consisting of walking, can assist counter this impact by maintaining lean muscle mass when you lose weight.

This can help in reducing the decrease in metabolic price that frequently occurs with weight loss, making your outcomes much easier to keep. What's even more, it can reduce age-related muscle loss, aiding you maintain more of your muscle mass toughness and also feature.

Recap: Walking can help stop some of the muscle loss that occurs when you drop weight. This assists minimize the drop in metabolic rate that takes place when you reduce weight, making the pounds much easier to keep off.

Walking Burns Belly Fat

Walking a lot of fat around your belly has actually been connected to an enhanced danger of illness like type 2 diabetic issues as well as cardiovascular disease. As a matter of fact, males with a midsection circumference greater than 40 inches (102 centimeters) as well as women with a midsection circumference higher than 35 inches (88 cm) have abdominal obesity, which is taken into consideration a health and wellness threat. Among the most reliable ways to lower stubborn belly fat is to frequently participate in cardio exercise, such as walking. In one small study, obese females that strolled for 50-- 70 minutes three times per week for 12 weeks, on average, minimized their waist area by 1.1 inches (2.8 cm) and also lost 1.5% of their body fat. An additional research discovered that people on a calorie-controlled diet who strolled for one hr five times per week for 12 weeks shed an additional 1.5 inches (3.7 centimeters) off their waists as well as 1.3% more body fat, contrasted to those who complied with the diet regimen alone. Various other research studies on the results of walking briskly for 30-- 60 minutes per day have observed similar outcomes.

Recap: On a regular basis taking part in moderate-intensity aerobic workout like strolling has been revealed to aid individuals lose stomach fat.

It Enhances Your Mood

Exercise is known to boost your state of mind. In fact, physical activity has actually been shown to boost your mood as well as reduce feelings of clinical depression, anxiousness and anxiety. It does this by making your brain more conscious the hormones serotonin and norepinephrine. These hormonal agents relieve feelings of clinical depression and also promote the launch of endorphins, which make you feel happy. This is a fantastic benefit by itself. However, experiencing an improvement in mood when you walk frequently might likewise make the practice less complicated to stay on par with. What's more, some studies have found that if you take pleasure in an exercise, it can boost the probability that you will certainly remain to do it. People often tend to work out less if they do not enjoy it, which can be an outcome of the workout being also physically requiring. This makes walking an outstanding selection, as it's a moderate-intensity workout. That's likely to inspire you to stroll more, as opposed to give up.

Recap: On a regular basis participating in exercise that you enjoy, such as strolling, can boost your mood and make you much more inspired to keep it up.

Walking Can Help You Maintain Weight Off

Many individuals who drop weight end up gaining it all back. However, normal workout plays an essential role in aiding you maintain weight-loss. Routine exercise like strolling does not just assist boost the quantity of power you melt day-to-day, however it also assists you construct more lean muscle mass so that you shed a lot more calories, even at rest. Moreover, joining normal, moderate-intensity exercise like walking can enhance your mood, making you most likely to remain active in the long-term. A current testimonial estimated that to preserve a stable weight, you need to stroll at the very least 150 mins per week. However, if you've shed a lot of weight, you may require to exercise greater than 200 mins weekly to stop on your own from reclaiming it. Actually, researches have located that individuals that work out the most are typically one of the most effective at keeping their weight loss, whereas individuals that exercise the least are likely to regain the weight. Integrating much more strolling into your day can aid you enhance the quantity of workout you contribute as well as do in the direction of your day-to-day activity objectives.

Recap: Staying energetic and relocating even more by walking throughout your day can help keep weight reduction. Exactly how to Incorporate More Walking Into Your Way of living Being much more literally energetic has a host of benefits, consisting of enhanced physical fitness and also mood, a reduced threat of disease and also a raised possibility of living a longer, healthier life.

As a result of this, it's recommended that individuals participate in a minimum of 150 minutes of moderate-intensity workout per week. In walking terms, that means walking for around 2.5 hours each week (at the very least 10 minutes at a time) at a quick rate. Doing even more workout than this has additional health and wellness advantages and also minimizes your risk of condition also better. There are numerous ways to boost the amount of walking you do and also achieve this target.

The complying with are some ideas:

- Utilize a physical fitness tracker and log your steps to motivate yourself to relocate more.

- Make a routine of taking a brisk walk on your lunch break or after dinner.

- Ask a buddy to join you for an evening walk.

- Walk your pet every day or join a friend on their pet strolls.

- Take a walking conference with an associate, rather than conference at your desk.

- Do errands like taking the kids to institution or mosting likely to the store walking.

- Walk to function. Park your car better away or obtain off your bus a couple of stops early as well as stroll the rest of the method if it's too far.

- Try choosing difficult as well as brand-new courses to keep your strolls interesting.

- Sign up with a walking group.

Every bit aids, so begin small and also attempt to progressively raise the quantity you walk daily.

RECAP: Including much more walking into your day can assist you burn extra calories as well as reduce weight.

The 10 Benefits of Regular Exercise

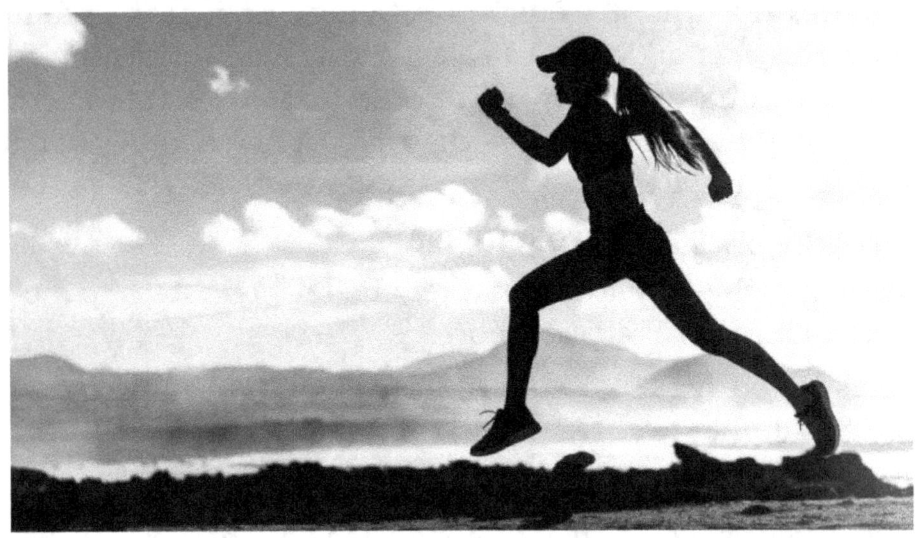

Workout is defined as any kind of activity that makes your muscular tissues work and requires your body to burn calories. There are many types of physical activity, consisting of swimming, running, jogging, walking as well as dancing, to name a few.

Being active has been shown to have lots of health and wellness advantages, both physically and psychologically. It may also aid you live longer.

Below are the leading 10 ways normal exercise benefits your body as well as brain.

1. It Can Make You Feel Happier

Exercise has been revealed to boost your mood and also decrease feelings of stress and anxiety, stress and also clinical depression. It produces modifications in the parts of the brain that regulate stress and stress and anxiety. It can additionally raise brain level of sensitivity for the hormones serotonin as well as norepinephrine, which alleviate feelings of clinical depression. In addition, workout can increase the manufacturing of endorphins, which are recognized to help create positive sensations and reduce the perception of pain. Moreover, exercise has actually been shown to minimize signs and symptoms in individuals dealing with anxiety. It can additionally help them be much more aware of their psychological state and also practice disturbance from their concerns. Interestingly, no matter how intense your exercise is. It seems that your mood can gain from workout no matter the intensity of the exercise.

In fact, a research study in 24 women that had actually been identified with anxiety showed that exercise of any type of intensity considerably lowered feelings of depression. The impacts of exercise on state of mind are so powerful that selecting to exercise (or otherwise) even makes a distinction over short periods. One research asked 26 healthy males and females that usually exercised regularly to either continue working out or stop exercising for two weeks. Those that quit exercising seasoned increases in negative state of mind.

Recap: Exercising consistently can improve your mood and lower feelings of anxiousness as well as clinical depression.

2. It Can Assist With Fat Burning

Some research studies have actually shown that inactivity is a significant consider weight gain and obesity. To comprehend the impact of exercise on weight reduction, it is necessary to comprehend the partnership between workout and also power expenditure. Your body spends energy in three methods: digesting food, preserving and also working out body features like your heartbeat as well as breathing.

While dieting, a minimized calorie consumption will decrease your metabolic rate, which will postpone weight management. On the other hand, routine exercise has actually been revealed to enhance your metabolic price, which will certainly burn more calories as well as aid you reduce weight. Additionally, researches have actually shown that incorporating aerobic workout with resistance training can maximize fat loss as well as muscle mass maintenance, which is vital for keeping the weight off

Recap: Exercise is important to sustaining a fast metabolic process and also melting more calories daily. It also aids you preserve your muscle mass and weight loss.

3. It Is Good for Your Muscles and Bones

Workout plays a crucial function in structure and also keeping strong muscular tissues and also bones. Exercise like weight training can stimulate bodybuilding when paired with appropriate protein intake. This is since workout assists launch hormones that promote the capacity of your muscle mass to absorb amino acids. This helps them expand and decreases their break down

As people age, they tend to shed muscle mass and feature, which can lead to injuries and impairments. Practicing regular exercise is essential to decreasing muscle loss as well as maintaining strength as you age. Likewise, exercise aids develop bone thickness when you're younger, in addition to helping avoid weakening of bones later in life. Remarkably, high-impact exercise, such as acrobatics or running, or odd-impact sports, such as soccer and basketball, have actually been revealed to advertise a greater bone density than non-impact sporting activities like swimming as well as cycling.

Recap: Physical activity aids you develop muscles as well as strong bones. It might likewise help stop weakening of bones.

4. It Can Enhance Your Energy Degrees

Workout can be a real power booster for healthy people, along with those experiencing various clinical problems. One study found that 6 weeks of routine workout minimized sensations of fatigue for 36 healthy individuals that had actually reported consistent exhaustion. In addition, workout can substantially raise power levels for individuals dealing with chronic fatigue syndrome (CFS) and also various other serious health problems.

As a matter of fact, exercise appears to be more effective at combating CFS than various other therapies, consisting of easy therapies like leisure and extending, or no treatment in all. Additionally, workout has actually been revealed to boost energy levels in individuals struggling with modern illnesses, such as cancer, HIV/AIDS as well as multiple sclerosis.

Recap: Engaging in routine exercise can raise your power levels. This holds true also in people with consistent tiredness as well as those suffering from serious diseases.

5. It Can Decrease Your Danger of Chronic Disease

Lack of routine physical activity is a main source of chronic disease. Routine exercise has been shown to boost insulin level of sensitivity, cardiovascular fitness and body composition, yet lower high blood pressure as well as blood fat levels. In contrast, a lack of normal exercise-- even in the short-term-- can bring about substantial boosts in stomach fat, which raises the threat of type 2 diabetes mellitus, heart disease and early death. Therefore, everyday physical activity is advised to minimize stubborn belly fat and decrease the threat of developing these diseases.

Recap: Daily exercise is vital to maintaining a healthy and balanced weight as well as lowering the threat of persistent condition.

6. It Can Assist Skin Wellness

Your skin can be impacted by the quantity of oxidative stress and anxiety in your body. When the body's antioxidant defenses can not completely repair the damage that complimentary radicals cause to cells, oxidative stress takes place. This can damage their interior frameworks and deteriorate your skin. Despite the fact that intense and also exhaustive exercise can add to oxidative damage, regular modest workout can boost your body's manufacturing of natural antioxidants, which help protect cells. Similarly, exercise can promote blood circulation and also cause skin cell adjustments that can assist delay the appearance of skin aging.

Recap: Moderate workout can provide antioxidant defense and promote blood circulation, which can shield your skin as well as hold-up signs of aging.

7. It Can Assist Your Brain Wellness and also Memory

Workout can improve mind feature and also protect memory as well as thinking skills. To begin with, it boosts your heart price, which advertises the flow of blood as well as oxygen to your brain. It can also boost the production of hormonal agents that can enhance the development of brain cells. Furthermore, the ability of workout to stop persistent illness can convert into advantages for your mind, considering that its feature can be impacted by these diseases. Normal physical activity is particularly essential in older adults since aging-- incorporated with oxidative anxiety and also inflammation-- advertises adjustments in mind structure and also function. Exercise has actually been shown to cause the hippocampus, a part of the mind that's essential for memory as well as discovering, to grow in size. This offers to boost mental feature in older adults. Lastly, workout has been revealed to reduce modifications in the brain that can cause Alzheimer's condition and also schizophrenia.

Recap: Normal workout improves blood circulation to the brain and also aids mind wellness as well as memory. Amongst older grownups, it can assist safeguard mental function.

8. It Can Assist With Leisure and also Rest Top Quality

Routine workout can aid you loosen up and also rest better. In regards to sleep quality, the energy exhaustion that takes place throughout exercise boosts recuperative processes throughout sleep. Moreover, the boost in body temperature that takes place during workout is thought to boost sleep top quality by assisting it go down during rest. Several research studies on the impacts of exercise on rest have gotten to similar conclusions. One research found that 150 mins of moderate-to-vigorous activity weekly can supply up to a 65% improvement in sleep quality. Another showed that 16 weeks of exercise increased sleep quality and assisted 17 people with sleeplessness sleep longer as well as more deeply than the control team. It likewise helped them really feel more energized during the day. What's even more, engaging in regular workout appears to be useful for the senior, that often tend to be influenced by sleep disorders. You can be adaptable with the kind of exercise you pick. It shows up that either cardio workout alone or aerobic workout integrated with resistance training can just as help rest high quality.

Recap: Normal physical activity, regardless of whether it is cardio or a combination of cardio as well as resistance training, can assist you sleep better and really feel even more energized throughout the day.

9. It Can Reduce Pain

Persistent discomfort can be devastating, yet exercise can actually help reduce it. Actually, for years, the suggestion for dealing with chronic pain was remainder and lack of exercise. Nevertheless, current studies show that workout aids alleviate persistent pain. An evaluation of numerous studies suggests that exercise helps participants with persistent pain lower their pain and boost their lifestyle. A number of research studies reveal that exercise can aid regulate discomfort that's related to numerous health problems, consisting of chronic low neck and back pain, fibromyalgia as well as chronic soft cells shoulder problem, among others. Additionally, physical activity can also elevate pain resistance and also reduce discomfort assumption.

Recap: Exercise has beneficial effects on the pain that's connected with different conditions. It can likewise boost discomfort tolerance.

10. It Can Promote a Much Better Sex Life

Exercise has been proven to improve libido. Taking part in regular exercise can enhance the cardiovascular system, improve blood flow, tone muscle mass as well as boost adaptability, all of which can improve your sex life. Physical activity can improve sex-related efficiency and also sexual pleasure, along with increase the frequency of sexual activity.

A team of ladies in their 40s observed that they experienced climaxes more frequently when they included more arduous workout, such as sprints, bootcamp and also weightlifting, right into their lifestyles. Likewise, amongst a group of

178 healthy men, the men that reported even more work-out hours per week had higher sexual feature scores. One research study discovered that a simple routine of a six-minute walk around your home assisted 41 males lower their erectile dysfunction symptoms by 71%.

Another research carried out in 78 inactive males disclosed how 60 minutes of walking each day (3 and a fifty percent days each week, usually) improved their sex-related behavior, including regularity, ample functioning and complete satisfaction. What's even more, a research demonstrated that women struggling with polycystic ovary disorder, which can decrease libido, increased their sex drive with regular resistance training for 16 weeks.

Recap: Exercise can assist boost sexual desire, feature and also performance in males and females. It can likewise aid lower the danger of erectile dysfunction in males.

CHAPTER4

Water Diet

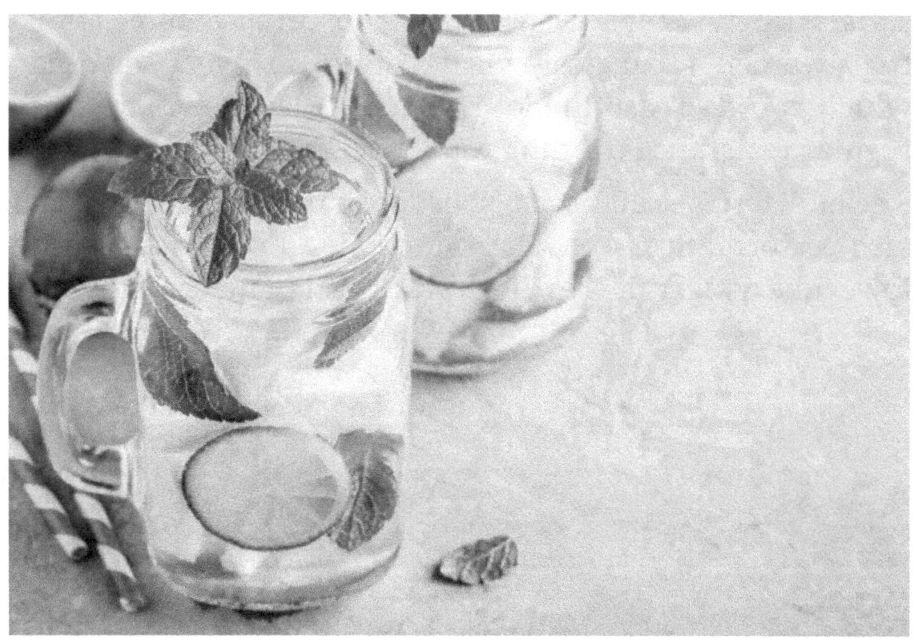

The Importance of Water in Your Diet Plan

Want a good diet tip? Drink more water.

onsuming lots of chilly, clear water is crucial for your health and, in fact, for your extremely survival. You can live much longer without food than you can without water. Water is an important part of all body features and also processes, consisting of food digestion and also removal. When you're on a diet regimen, water additionally functions as a weight-loss aid due to the fact that it can assist you consume less.

Drinking water is important throughout fat burning due to the fact that it supplies hydration without unwanted calories. Consuming alcohol non-caloric fluids like water prior to or with a meal can help a dieter really feel full faster," clarifies Donna Logan, RD, a signed up dietitian at the University of Texas Medical School in Houston. "So in addition to not adding calories, drinking water may help replace or avoid unnecessary food calories found in snacks or additional portions at mealtime. Drinking water also assists flush wastes from the body, which is especially important throughout times of fat metabolism as well as weight-loss."

Water: Drinking Sufficient to Boost Your Diet

Suggestions from the Food and also Nourishment Board are for women to get 91 ounces per day and men 125 ounces from all sources-- water, other beverages, and also foods with a high water content.

When it comes to water alone, discusses Logan, "A general suggestion is to consume eight 8-ounce mugs of water per day, for an overall of 64 ounces. This is a generalization only, and also actual fluid demands are affected by diet regimen, exercise, body composition, and environment."

As an example, this number goes up if you work out-- a

key to effective weight loss-- and also much more so in heat when it's feasible to lose regarding the equivalent of a quart of water in an hour, according to the American Council on Workout. You'll wish to consume alcohol water prior to, during, as well as after every exercise.

Don't wait to really feel parched to start drinking-- that's a sign that dehydration has actually currently begun to occur. You intend to consume water throughout the day, on a regular basis.

Water:

Four Tips for Getting Your Fill up

Below are some simple tricks for getting sufficient water while weight loss:

Use a water tracker:

A water tracker is simply a device which aids you keep an eye on how much water you consume alcohol. A water tracker can offer a visuals document of 8 glasses of water which are checked off as they are eaten. For instance, consuming alcohol a 20-ounce container of water would equate into 2 as well as a fifty percent cups on the tracker. Such trackers are offered online or can be quickly replicated," explains Logan.

Add water throughout your day:

Individuals can utilize a variety of techniques to help guarantee they get enough water. Some lug a 64-ounce container of water as well as beverage throughout the day, with the objective of consuming all the water before they go to bed. Those who hang out away from residence might take a mobile 16-ounce container, recognizing that they need to load and drink it four times throughout the day. Others connect drinking with routine activities throughout the day, such as alcohol consumption fluid at dishes, prior to cleaning their teeth, or after feeding the dogs, claims Logan.

Obtain water via food:

Vegetables as well as fruits, particularly those that are fresh and juicy, give fluid to the diet plan. Like water, clear soups as well as broths aid dieters really feel full for really few calories, adding to fat burning. However, beware of creamy soups that, while adding fluids, include many calories. Skim milk, and also no-added and low-fat sugar yogurts as well as puddings likewise aid hydration as well as nutrition without extreme calories," suggests Logan. Melons and citrus fruits additionally have a really high water content.

Jazz up your water glass:

Many individuals discover that adding low- or non-caloric flavors to water, such as a wedge of fruit, assists please their appetite cravings," adds Logan. This is likewise a really inexpensive method to make your very own flavorful water.

If you desire your diet to function, you need to consume a lot of water. Water can load you up, decrease your appetite, and aid your body eliminate waste from that fat you're burning. So what are you waiting on? Water is readily available right now from your tap, as well as it's totally free.

10 DAY WATER FAST

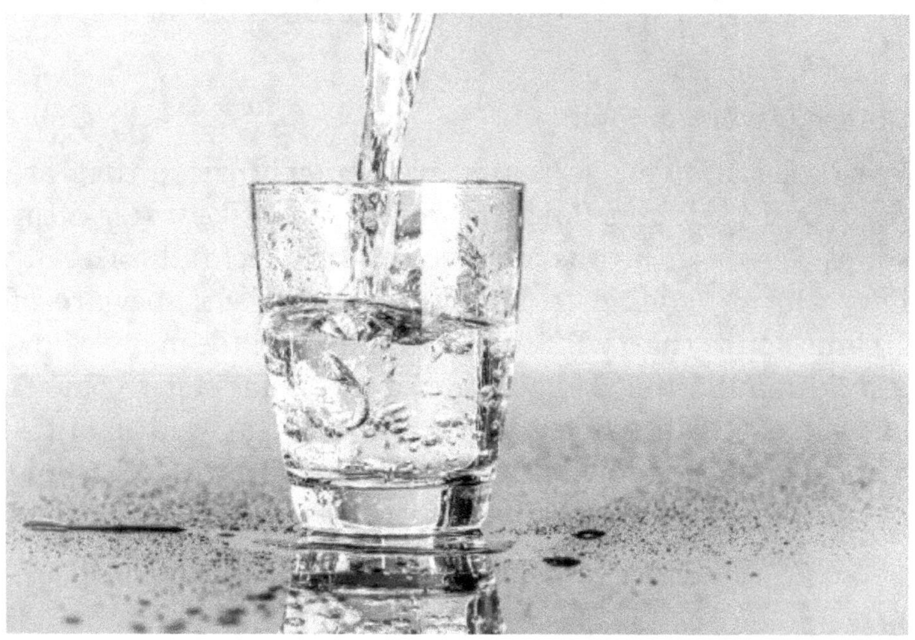

Why Do a 10 Day Fast?

-Anti-Cancer: Leveraging the metabolic theory of cancer cells as well as Dr. Thomas Seyfried's job, fasting might be an effective technique to minimize our future threat of cancer.

-Body Immune System Performance: Cyclic fasting has been shown to regrow immune system cells which weaken 'naturally' as we age or using environmental or various other disrespects. Hence, it may stave or minimize off a few of this natural degeneration as well as maintain us much healthier.

-A More Powerful Body: Lean body mass gains including bone density increase and also muscular tissue mass rise have actually additionally been tracked in research studies and myself.

-Body Fat Elimination: Fasting or cycles of fasting can be a valuable method for eliminating unwanted excess body fat.

Wellness benefits!

Have you experienced the wellness benefits of consuming even more water? Such as even more energy, clear emphasis, as well as better digestion? Well, I took it an action further as well as after Christmas this past year, I attempted water fasting for 10 days-- 10 DAYS! Was it due to the fact that there was a lot exceptional food over the holidays that my body could not digest all that remained in it? No. Did I expand a big bulge on my back (like a camel), that enabled me to indulge off of its fat books? Nope. Was I starving? Definitely for the very first 3 days, yet then not a lot.

You see, several months prior, my other half and I chose to quick as a way of purifying our bodies and giving our gastrointestinal track a chance to rest and also heal itself. We had actually never tried such a feat prior to and heard mixed testimonials regarding fasting, yet we figured it couldn't harm to give it a try.

WHY WATER FASTING?

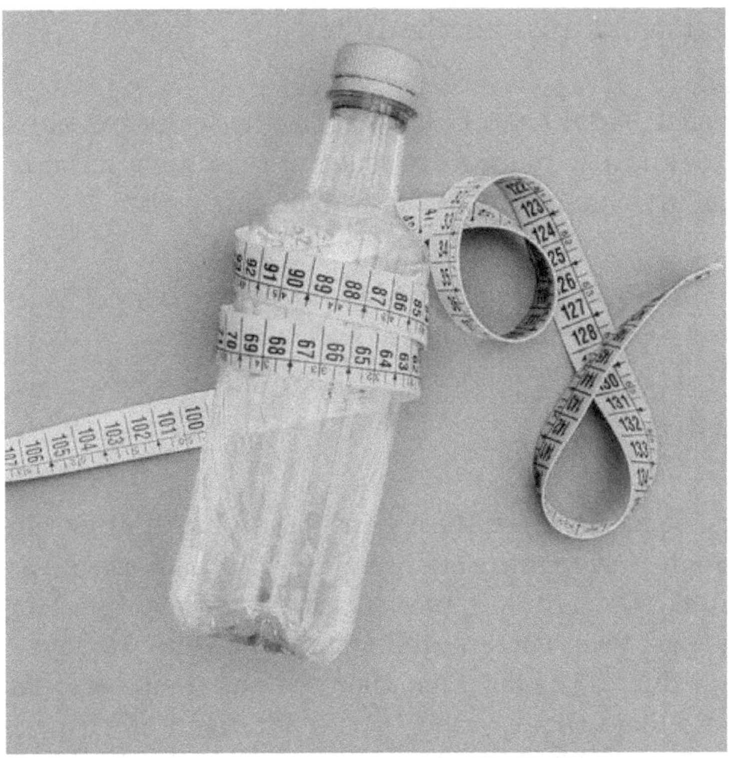

A few years ago I had the enjoyment of working with a gentleman from Europe that wasn't also far from his 60th birthday. We discussed a range of topics: financing, business economics, health, nutrition ... practically whatever under the sun. His sights were so hugely various than mine (clearly because he was from another country), yet speaking with him assisted to expand my own horizons on the various subjects.

Among them was water fasting.

One mid-day he shared that twenty years ago, he was diagnosed with late phase prostate cancer cells. He was in outstanding wellness, was an energetic cyclist and ate a mainly vegan diet plan. Yet he had cancer. His oncologist at the time had actually recommended numerous treatments, varying from chemotherapy and radiation, to surgical procedure, as well as even the removal of the prostate. My colleague wasn't sold on the suggestions of the oncologist, so he considered different approaches of treating as well as also perhaps healing the cancer cells. One of those methods was water fasting. Versus the guidance of his medical professional, he was figured out to combat his cancer naturally. He started water fasting for 40 days, taking in no food and also absolutely nothing to consume besides water. Now around 18 years from his original diagnosis, his cancer cells remains in remission and he lives a quite typical life. So what transformed? He integrated water fasting right into his way of life, permanently.

By regularly as well as regularly completing long water fasts and also permanently transforming his diet regimen to consist of more wholesome, nutrient dense foods, he currently lives a much healthier life. To monitor his fasts and also the experience as well as results, he maintains a water fasting log.

MY CHOICE TO TRY WATER FASTING

Interested and also doubtful at the time, I started combing the internet to validate his attraction as well as love of fasting. Post after write-up, page after web page was filled with testimonies of people that like fasting. They raved regarding the health and wellness benefits, spiritual benefits and so forth. You'll even find that some proclaim fasting will certainly cure cancer, HIV/Aids, acne, anxiety as well as fibromyalgia. Whether this information holds true, I have no suggestion.

Despite all the nitty gritty details that the internet will certainly generate, my friend revealed me to something I believed I'd never ever attempt: water fasting. Promptly after looking into the advantages, I strongly declared to my partner, "I'M GOING ON A 7 DAY WATER QUICKLY!"

She assumed I was crazy.

No, I didn't have cancer cells. And in truth, I just wished to try it since the advantages seemed excellent as well as there were virtually no risks. To reduce into the water quick, I initially started with the master cleanse. According to United States News, the master clean contains water, newly squeeze lemons, cayenne pepper and syrup. You consume 6-10 glasses a day for at least 10 days, and include a natural laxative tea during the night.

I honestly found this method undesirable.

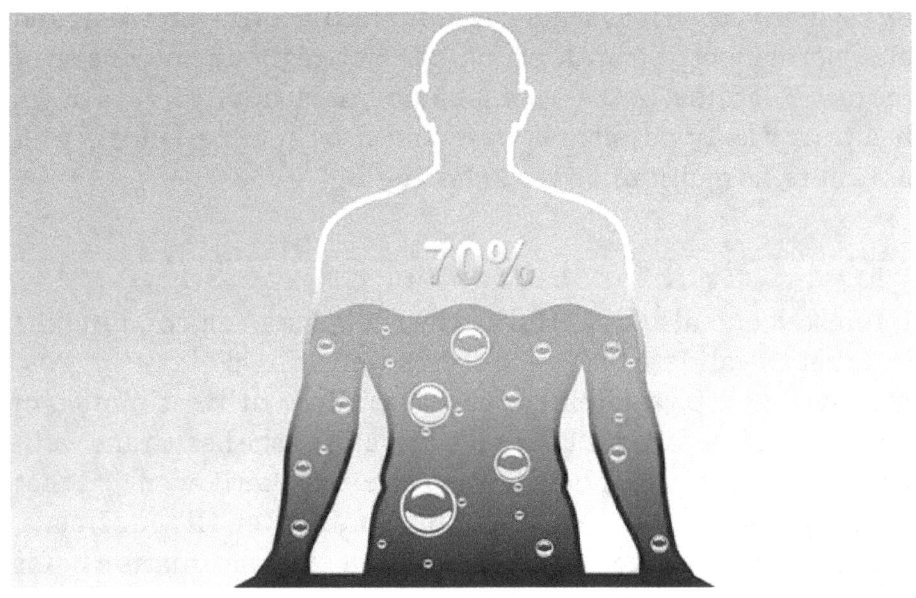

While some enjoy the taste of this concoction, the chili pepper made me gag and also the laxative tea had me up at 3am. My initial effort at not eating lasted 3 days prior to enjoying a burrito from a local taco shop.Fast forward a couple of years and the concept of water fasting resurfaced between my better half and also myself and also we both chose to fast after the holidays. My plan was a 7-10 day water quick while hers was a customized 5 day healthy smoothie quick.

I selected water fasting for a number of reasons:

Water fasts are typically the quickest way to detox. Some also consider this the only "genuine" means to purify your body and also bring it back in check.

Water fasts are the most hard. I thought if I might go ten days on water alone, all future fasts of juice or smoothies would be very easy in comparison.

WELLNESS ADVANTAGES OF WATER FASTING

There are a number of benefits to drinking water generally. As well as in my study of the wellness advantages of water fasting, I discovered many write-ups. Some were supported by study, as well as some were not. I summarized my searchings for below, however if you choose to see the research study for yourself, I suggest checking out "Water Fasting for Health." It's a very practical book with lots of research write-ups on the topic of water fasting.

For a doctor's viewpoint of water fasting, "Fasting and also Eating for Health" would certainly be my leading choice.

FAT BURN

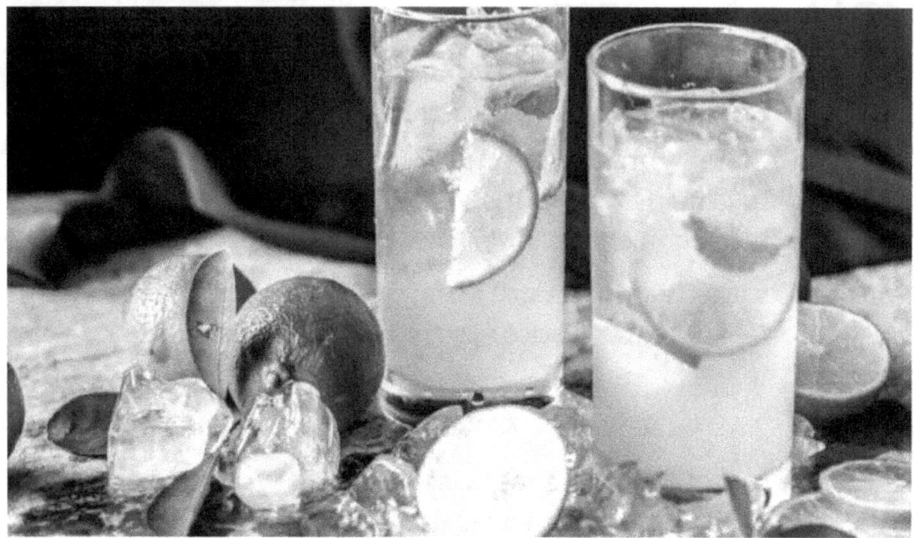

After your body has actually used all the excess calories, it starts melting fat. By default, when you melt fat, you lose weight. Not eating simply to lose weight is a very disputed topic. You must be EXCEPTIONALLY mindful when you return to eating since your metabolic rate slows down to a crawl. Otherwise the weight will certainly come right back.Nevertheless, if food is reestablished correctly as well as in small amounts, keeping the weight off is possible.

Keep in mind: My wife and I reduced weight merely by switching to a whole foods diet plan. If you're attempting to drop weight, I extremely recommend transforming your eating routines as opposed to water fasting.

HYPERTENSION

This was among the primary factors I selected to finish a fast this year. My high blood pressure had been approaching in the direction of the 130/80 array, often a little greater. Fasting promptly brought it down to the 115/70 array. It rises and fall depending upon the day, however bringing it down 15 factors behaved!

PSYCHOLOGICAL CLARITY

This is probably a side effect of your body not working extremely hard and also consequently triggering immense leisure, but you have the ability to think much more clearly when not eating compared to regular eating behaviors. Choices were simple to make and "difficult" situations were a lot more workable. I discovered that fasting aided me to place points in point of view.

VISION

Yes, your vision can sharpen! An odd, however pleasurable negative effects. It doesn't suggest you can quit wearing your get in touches with or toss your glasses in the trash bin, but it's possible for your eyes to function a lot more efficiently.

CANCER PREVENTION

A 2008 research study at the College of The golden state at Berkeley discovered that eating every other day reduced the price at which cells generated, an effect understood to decrease the growth of cancers cells. In animal versions, intermittent fasting was found to decrease cancer development on the skin and also in bust cells. If fasting has the potential to deal with and even possibly cure cancer cells, why isn't this being assessed regularly as opposed to the most recent and best drug?

LIVE LONGER

It's hard to explain the scientific research behind this, but research study reveals that those that quickly live much longer. Does simply going without consuming extend life? Possibly not. My guess would be the continual removal of toxins and also permitting the body to relax from its everyday job.

DETOXIFY

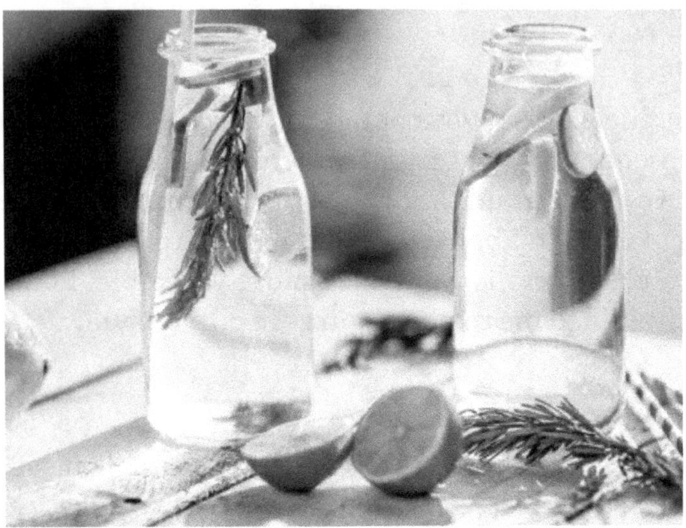

Isn't this the new trend? Individuals throughout the world are getting on the "let's detoxification as well as be healthy and balanced" bandwagon, screaming for their food to be devoid of Pesticides and gmos. What these individuals do not realize is that their "craze" is reality-- fasting enables the body to rid itself of contaminants. Introducing and preserving a proper diet full of real and healthy food truly is much better for you.

Keep in mind: Now that my fast is over, I do not wish to fall back right into bad practices. To routinely cleanse my body from the periodic splurge, I include detox healthy smoothies and detox bathrooms into my weekly regimen.

DIGESTIVE SYSTEM FUNCTION

Your digestion system will love you for fasting. It takes about 3 days into the rapid for your system to entirely close down. Fluids in, fluid out. After breaking the fast (securely as well as carefully naturally), you'll locate that your defecation act as if they're on steroids.

WHEN WATER FASTING, water HIGH QUALITY

My father was a plumbing technician as well as he was constantly very particular concerning the high quality of water we consumed. A part of his problem still runs through me, and also the high quality of your water deserves stating if it's all you'll be drinking for a period of time. Berkey water filters are the best of the best, known for taking arsenic, uranium, aluminum as well as fluoride out of normal tap water. While it's on the more expensive side, it's absolutely worth taking into consideration not just for water fasting, but for enhancing the water in your house in its entirety. Consider an infuser water container if you're not a huge water enthusiast in the very first place as well as you don't assume water tastes good. You can add pieces of fruit that will taste the water, making it extra palatable. There are infuser water pitchers as well, for making bigger batches of flavorful water. My favorite flavor combination is cucumber + mint + lemon.

MY EXPERIENCE WITH WATER FASTING FOR 10 DAYS

Days 1-3

The first few days were rough.

It was throughout this time that the detoxifying signs were the most awful. There was hunger, headache … it was rough. I am a coffee enthusiast and absolutely nothing beats pouring a warm mug of fresh made coffee right into a ceramic mug, drinking the java goodness before starting the day. I attribute the pure anguish of days 1-3 to high levels of caffeine withdrawal. At the same time, Mrs. Crumbs food preparation dinner for the children as well as knowing I couldn't consume was ruthless.

Days 4-6

Nowadays were reasonably easy.

By this time my gastrointestinal system had actually shut down and the cravings pains had gone away. My tongue was commonly covered with a thick white movie. This is obviously normal and also an additional detoxing signs and symptom. I started losing weight, 1-- 1 1/2 pounds per day, yet there was no worry mosting likely to function, playing guitar at church or executing any other daily physical functions.

Day 7

I will never forget this particular day-- ever. This was the most miserable day I have actually ever before lived on world earth. I returned from work sensation excellent, not starving, thinking plainly. And after that my life was flipped upside-down. My remarkable wife pulled a newly baked loaf of rosemary olive oil bread from the oven. I was immediately angry and also I wanted that bread. However it had not been even feasible at this point. When your gastrointestinal system closes down around day 3, it takes a few days to bring it back up to speed up. You do this by extremely slowly introducing food to your digestive system ... alcohol consumption juice for 1-2 days, fresh fruit for another couple days, fit to be tied veggies for another day or two. The procedure of reintroducing food can take anywhere from 7-14 days prior to your gastrointestinal system back up to totally functional. Consuming any kind of solid food while in a fasted state can bring about severe pain as well as even a hospital stay!

Day 8-10

These days were virtually an exact replica of days 4-6. By the end of day 10, I had actually lost 15 pounds and was ready to eat again.

WATER FASTING: ALL-TIME LOW LINE

Overall, I enjoyed water fasting. It was testing, yet the health and wellness benefits were well worth it. My digestion boosted, high blood pressure was reduced as well as I may have lowered the opportunity of obtaining cancer cells. I intend on doing it again later this year, and also probably continue to fast at the very least one or two times a year from now on. My partner likes food excessive to do a water quickly, be she's dedicated to doing a shake fast with me whenever I water quick. If the idea of water fasting is a little bit difficult, that could be a choice for you!

NOT EATING As Well As CLEANSING ON A REGULAR BASIS

Water fasting is on the much more severe side of detoxing your body. However, there are lots of other means to detox on a regular basis to maintain your body functions optimal. DIY Apple Cider Vinegar Potion is terrific for an everyday increase to your gastro-intestinal and immune system.

A Detoxification Bathroom is a simple means to kick back and enable your body to recover from the daily toxic substances we run into. Consuming Alcohol a Detoxification Smoothie every now and then will enhance your body systems as well as maintain it running smoothly.

Do It Yourself Detoxification Face Mask with Charcoal and Clay assists to remove your skin and enhance your skin. Using a Detoxifying Salt Scrub is a wonderful method to cleanse your skin and also scrub while eliminating contaminants.

Day-to-day Detox and No Excuses Detoxification are recipe books each with 100 recipes for healthy and balanced eating. Real food consuming as well as detoxing with diet regimen is an exceptional method to maintain your body free from toxic substances.

Numerous of those detox approaches make use of Bentonite Clay. It's so helpful for your body in several methods, if you're simply starting out try one of these smaller sized containers of Bentonite Clay.. But if you resemble me as well as utilize it for all type of things around the house, buy it in bulk!